MW00935468

Doctor with M.E.

My journey with

"Chronic Fatigue Syndrome"

Dr. K.N. Hng

Copyright © 2019 Andrew Alexander Roger Brown
All Rights Reserved

No material appearing in this book may be modified, reproduced or transmitted in any form or medium or by any means without written permission from the copyright owner.

ISBN: 9781796715460

Disclaimer:

This is not a medical textbook.

This is not a complete guide to ME/CFS.

This book does not make recommendations on tests or treatments.

This book does not replace proper assessment by a qualified doctor.

No warranty is given that the information provided within this book is accurate, up to date, or unambiguous.

The author and publisher take no responsibility for any actions taken after reading this book.

Get in touch, purchase our album,

or collaborate on medical education:

RColourMusic@hotmail.com

Facebook group:

Dr Hng's ME/CFS Friends – all welcome!

(group rules apply)

**https://www.facebook.com/groups/
drhngsfriends/**

Twitter:

Dr Hng's Friends @DoctorwithME

Give this book to your doctor with this letter!

http://bit.ly/DrHngLetter-w-Book

Free handout for health care professionals:

**http://bit.ly/Introduction
ToMEbyDrHng**

PLEASE donate for medical education:

Dr Hng's M.E. Education and Research Fund CIC

The Royal Bank of Scotland

Sort code: 83-04-25

Account number: 19374150

IBAN: GB76RBOS83042519374150

SWIFT BIC: RBOSGB2L

My photos:

http://bit.ly/DrHngPhotos

Dedication

This book is dedicated to all ME/CFS sufferers, a misunderstood, neglected and forgotten group of patients, many of whom have died in the absence of the help they needed, and/or suffered further damage from incorrect, harmful treatments.

This YouTube video makes a beautiful dedication:

**http://bit.ly/MEandMe
Dedication**

Preface

I have a story to tell. There are many things in here which I am not at all comfortable sharing, yet I want to tell the whole story. Therefore I have decided to share them. I hope doing so will help educate, inform, and raise awareness. From my own experience, both as a doctor and then as a patient, this condition is poorly understood. After all, isn't *everyone* tired all the time?

CONTENTS

Not Good Enough

I was a doctor. A busy, National Health Service, very senior Junior Doctor. Then I fell ill with Myalgic Encephalomyelitis, also known as Chronic Fatigue Syndrome.

I was struggling desperately for months, even years. Failing to perform at work, being told I was slow in clinic, that I wasn't showing leadership, that I didn't carry myself like a Consultant, etc. I was just so exhausted all the time, I barely managed to do the minimum. I drank more, and more, and MORE coffee, squeezing every last ounce of energy out of my poor tired body.

For being "not good enough", I got more things thrown at me. More work-based assessments, more appraisals, more meetings, more portfolio activity, in addition to the usual courses, fifteen-hundred-word assignments, and teaching presentations to prepare. This only added to my load.

So I tried harder. Soooo hard. Staying up late every night working on all that was asked, fighting sleep. Investing hours into teaching activities, and speeding through clinics. Working relentlessly through the grueling 12.5 hour Long Day and Long Night shifts, pushing through the exhaustion.

I clocked up as many as nine patients in a clinic, dosed up on coffee and running on sheer willpower. When a Consultant suddenly took ill (and sadly never returned), I took on and managed extra clinics on my own.

Yet no matter what I did, it was never enough. My training time was extended as I had not proven myself able to take on the heavy workload and responsibilities of a Consultant.

A Desperate Struggle

One night shift I could not get up off the chair in the office. All night. My whole body had turned to lead, an enormous weight. A mighty magnet pulled every part of my body flat down against the desk, seat and floor. All I could do was answer questions from the neglected first year doctor, left alone out on the shop floor. With great difficulty, forcing my head and arms to move and work the telephone.

That was flagged up. It was serious. And I took desperate measures. Like paying for a hotel when on Nights just to try to sleep and perform better, and my child frequently missing her bath to reduce the strain. My boss referred me for hypnotherapy.

In desperation, I took myself to see the Occupational Health doctor. For the first time I was able to express how I struggled, yet failed. A fact that so far had to be hidden, in my efforts to prove myself capable. I dissolved into tears.

~~~~~~~

Following that visit, I was commenced on an antidepressant. And then had to deal with terrible side effects. Now on top of everything else, I suffered severe constipation and juggled insane amounts of time in the toilet, feeling permanently bloated, gaining weight and draining my time and energy even further. (sobs!)

My shifts were cut back slightly, but I didn't improve. It just slowed my decline. After a Long Day (12.5 hrs), I would be absolutely shattered all the next day, which I accepted as normal. But on the second and third days, I still felt exactly the same, as if I had been on-call the day before.

I was in constant mild pain. All my muscles were stiff

and every movement ached, as if I had run a marathon the previous day. This got much worse after every on-call shift, and for days afterwards every movement would be a test of will against pain and exhaustion. And still I didn't know I was ill.

On the fourth and fifth days I would feel only a tiny bit better. I still fought exhaustion, ached, and struggled to excel. When the next on-call shift came around, I hadn't yet recovered. At the end of one shift I must have looked ghastly, for a colleague exclaimed when he saw me, "Now that's a broken woman!"

~~~~~~~

Getting up in the morning required superhuman effort. I began to set my alarm to an earlier time to give myself longer to get ready. I wasn't safe driving. Not only did I fall asleep driving home from work, I struggled to keep awake driving in. The 1.5 hour commute made things worse. A "short day" would be 12 hours long. I was constantly worried that I would die in a car crash and leave my children orphaned.

Once home, I would collapse onto the couch for half an hour or more. This upset my children, who had been looking forward to seeing me, so my husband and I determined that I should park up somewhere and rest in the car before returning to the house. I deteriorated further, and then I was sleeping in the car park at the hospital before driving home, for I could not face the journey.

After Long Days, as badly as I needed it, I was too exhausted to manage a shower. A change of clothes had to do.

It's Not Depression!

On the 29th of June 2016, six months after that fateful night shift, I could not carry on any longer. I will never forget that day. I went to my GP, burst into tears again, and cried, "I don't feel safe!" I knew if I carried on I'd kill somebody.

Sobbing uncontrollably again earned me yet another anti-depressant. This time it made me stop eating, and I became very weak as a result. When I realised what had happened, I threw the rest out. I couldn't afford to be made even more ill, and I was still reeling from the side effects of the last one!

With the first anti-depressant, I had persevered for over two months, knowing it takes time to have an effect. I didn't feel depressed, but I was so desperate for an explanation, for someone to know what to do, I was willing to consider anything. And it gave me a truly horrid experience, whilst also fighting my losing battle at work. Even after discontinuing the tablets, it was many months before I was less bloated, and a total of six months before I felt properly back to normal. The constipation had been so severe, it really seemed as though my bowels had seized up completely and I was literally carrying around that much backlog! Days would pass without me need-ing the toilet. When I did go, the urge was half-hearted, and it would be a long, difficult, energy-draining exercise I could ill afford.

I never felt depressed, even with all that I was going through. I have always had a positive outlook on life, with a tendency to err on the side of optimism. At work, I never doubted I could succeed and become a Consultant, despite everything. Even at home, lying on the sofa with my eyes shut because I was so ill, I was happy. I delighted in the precious sound of my children playing, and felt so glad to be resting at last!

I was finally diagnosed at the specialist CFS/ME clinic. They confirmed I wasn't depressed. I was thoroughly screened for depression, anxiety and sleep apnoea, scoring near zero for all of them. The specialist said, "Just because you cry doesn't mean you're depressed."

Mild − significant reduction in activity

Moderate − approximately 50% reduction in activity

Severe − mostly housebound

Very severe − mostly bedridden and may need help with basic functions †

† 2012 International Consensus Primer
Full reference on pg.114

Run into the Ground

Life was UTTER HELL before I went off sick. I wanted so desperately to stay home and sleep, yet I had no "reason" to be off work, no "illness", and there wasn't anything obviously wrong with me. Just being exhausted was not an acceptable reason. Instead, it was the accepted norm!

As a doctor, you work the rotas, relentless and unsustainable as they are. AND sit exams, maintain your portfolio, attend courses, prepare teaching resources, and undertake extra projects such as audit, quality improvement, or write up research for publication, all in your own time, just to prove yourself competent and employable at the end of your training. Meanwhile the rotas become more and more punishing, as staffing levels drop unmanageably due to changes in government policy. Being exhausted is therefore just normal.

At the end of 2013, I returned to work following a prolonged absence on sick leave and maternity leave. I failed miserably. My supervisor asked me, "What's wrong with you?" but I didn't have an answer for him. I never let him know how I struggled to stay awake in clinic, sometimes even whilst speaking to a patient. I believed I was simply "unfit" after my prolonged absence. I was so ashamed of it, I was unable to share the secret.

That was the start of the escalating doses of coffee.

Over the next two years, my performance and competence improved significantly, with sheer determination and grit. I needed little supervision, I excelled at teaching, and my specialist knowledge increased steadily. I received brilliant patient feedback and got many competencies signed off.

But I did not shine. It took all I had to execute the work. I did not have the energy to lead, nor the strength to rise to Consultant level performance. I was so exhausted, I didn't even have the energy to smile at people.

In the end, I ran myself into the ground. I worked to the point of collapse, vainly trying to be the super-woman that doctors who dare to have children are required to be. The situation was extreme beyond belief. I was forced to neglect my own physical needs, I self-medicated with sedatives in order to sleep at unnatural hours when on Nights, and I barely saw my children.

That night when I was unable to function, I should have alerted the supervising Consultant, who was home in bed after a very long day herself. But what was I to say? That I was tired? Besides, I wasn't planning to stay in the office all night. "Just ten more minutes," I told myself. "I WILL get up."

Not understanding that I was actually very sick, I

fought on. I had collapsed but could not admit it. I believed I would be able to push myself back onto my feet after a little rest. I saw no other option.

The sad fact is that being a doctor in the National Health Service is so demanding that I couldn't even recognise I was ill. Exhaustion just seemed normal. Instead of seeking help, I felt ashamed, and just pushed myself harder. "Helpful" appraisals and recommendations aimed at improving my perfor-mance just added to my load, my supervisors also failing to notice that I was ill.

For all of us in the NHS, seeing a colleague look exhausted is a normal daily occurrence. We all feel that way ourselves on a regular basis, and we can't offer much support, as we are all stretched to the limit. We don't listen to our bodies – we don't have the option to. If we did, the service would collapse and God forbid, the government would have to increase spending on staffing levels!

Living with ME

I am nearly totally housebound. I cannot drive or take a stroll along my street. I very rarely leave the house and every excursion costs me dearly.

I have minimal energy and do little more than just watch TV or sit at the computer, eat, and nap. Each day I manage just one task – if I fold some laundry, I do nothing else that day. I only have a shower every four, five, or even seven days. My hair only gets washed when it is actually disgusting, and I brush my teeth just once each day, with the help of an electric toothbrush. When energy is spent, I cannot even watch TV, for following a plot is too much work. Every afternoon I spend hours in bed.

All other housework is impossible. I cannot care for my children. I cannot take them to school. I used to make an effort to wash them, but then at my first therapy session at the specialist clinic, I realised that I was having to choose between bathing my children and having my own shower. The realisation brought painful tears, again. Life was just such a losing battle!

The fatigue is absolutely debilitating. It is more than just feeling lacklustre. It is an all-consuming feeling of the body, head and limbs having turned into lead, and carrying the weight of stone. When gripped by it, it is a struggle even to move a finger, or to speak. So you can't call or text a friend. You suffer alone.

At other times I simply feel exhausted, having done only an hour or less of very light activity. All my muscles are sore and I am overcome by an over-whelming need to lie down and shut my eyes. Many times I have fallen asleep, leaving the children to their own devices.

I move slowly. Sometimes VERY slowly. I am stiff and ache all over. Apparently this is because my muscles do not have the ATP molecules required to clear away the lactic acid build-up from even the minimal activity that I do. Any over-exertion results in a crash. Then my muscle pains become even more pronounced, and my joints stiffen too. For days I feel horribly sick, and I am stuck in bed for hours on end, not having the strength to get up. At particularly bad times my joints seize up altogether. Then even shifting my weight becomes laboured torture, all of me as stiff as a piece of wood. When the stiffness and heaviness overwhelms, I crawl on the floor, step after painful step.

~~~~~~~

When my pre-schooler was referred to the Clumsy Children's Clinic for an unusual number of falls and bruises, I tried to see if her heel-toe walk had improved from her first attempt at the doctor's surgery. I got up to show her what to do, and was shocked to discover I was even more unsteady than she was, completely unable to execute the walk! With a sinking feeling, I realised that my wide based gait isn't just because of general weakness and stiffness, but is due to the neurological consequences of the disease. (sobs, again.)

~~~~~~~

After my daily naps I wake paralysed, stuck in the netherworld between wakefulness and sleep, completely unable to move. My eyes stay shut and my body stays still. I am mentally submerged under ten feet of water – my own Netherland.

Beyond ten feet down, the water is completely murky and impenetrable. I am asleep. At just under ten feet, there appears a vague awareness of the outside world. Here I drift, near the bottom, sometimes sinking back again into oblivion.

Very slowly, I drift up out of the depths. I become

more and more aware of sounds and where I am as I rise, but until I reach shallow areas, complex thoughts do not penetrate and I remain completely paralysed, my body feeling like a dead weight.

Meanwhile, my heart starts pounding uncomfortably. It is as if it's the engine that powers the process of waking up, for this happens every time. It carries on for a long period, often until after I am out of bed. When thoughts eventually penetrate, I am mostly wishing the pounding palpitations will stop.

When I reach the surface, I can finally open my eyes, and properly process sensory input from the outside world. I can't tell you how long I am stuck in the netherworld. I am not able to look at the clock until I am out of it.

Once my mind is out of Netherland, I must wait for the stone weight to lift from my body. I might be able to turn in bed, but it is another hour before I can get out of bed, and for a further hour or two, I can do no more than just sit in a chair, struggling to move even an arm. If I try to get up too soon, I discover how heavy my body is still, and fall back into bed again.

I am also hypersensitive. I must keep my eyes shaded and my earplugs in place while I wait for the rest of my strength to return. Gradually, light and sound becomes less and less uncomfortable until eventually, I am able to handle them and remove my protections. Sometimes this takes longer, and I keep my sunglasses on, or baseball cap placed low, after I am up.

~~~~~~~

The specialist clinic calls this the Slow Start. Other symptoms include sudden near-fainting spells on standing, ventricular ectopics (a type of palpitations that has been recorded on tape), frequent sore throats with painful lymph glands, and multiple other infections. I am unable to stand for more than two minutes at a time. At best I can manage five minutes. Any longer is torture.

I also get fasciculations. This is when a small piece of muscle randomly decides to take on a life of its own and do a little jig. This lasts minutes or happens repeatedly, which is extremely distracting.

Some patients describe severe intolerance to light and sound, which causes them agonising headaches. I often feel an uncomfortable glare even in very low levels of light, and stripes or high contrast patterns create and intolerable sensory assault. I keep a pair of sunglasses and ear plugs with me, indoors and out, just in case.

If anybody talks, watches videos or listens to music in the same room, I find it impossible to concentrate on my work. The cognitive load is simply too great.

Sound demands too much brainpower, stopping all other cognitions in their tracks. Even a distant lawnmower renders any work impossible. To be productive at the computer, I must don drab, dark coloured, monotone clothing. The contrast of my own socks, my skin, or a different coloured item on the table against the rest of my surroundings can make it impossible to focus.

My brain only has one single working track, and a slow one at that. If that track is occupied with processing other sensory input, nothing else is possible. Such is life with my miniscule rate of energy production. I am not in the slow lane. I am not even on the road. I am the snail creeping alongside, in the grass.

~~~~~~~

When I am tired, I develop word-finding difficulties. Words get replaced with variably (or not!) related ones. One morning "glass" became "paper".

It's not that I don't know the right words. I do, and I find them within seconds when I stop and concentrate. However, during speech they do not come quickly enough and others take their place. This normally automatic process becomes hard work, as if my brain functions cease when energy is in short supply. That morning I settled for "window". "Glass" would have come if I had tried harder, but "window" did the job.

Typing brings its own challenges. As a touch typist, words are produced as I think them. But as I type, words get dropped, and I am not aware of it until I go back and check what I have typed. The word substitutions occur as well and again, I am completely unaware of it. Once, "top left" became "top right". Not only had my brain substituted a word for something else in the same category, it had also substituted its commands to my hands, so that the wrong word was executed, completely unbeknownst to me! How can I think "left", type "right", and still believe I typed "left"?!

My husband answered the question that night.
"Because you're not doing it with a typewriter, but a type lefter," he said.
"What?" I asked, uncomprehending.
Then I thought no more of it, and settled down to sleep. Ten seconds later, I chuckled. My brain had continued processing the joke, and got there eventually – at ME speed!

Unfortunately, related words often have opposite meanings. Imagine trying to write and edit a book!

~ ~ ~ ~ ~ ~ ~

Reading is a real struggle. I can read leaflets, and just about manage single articles if they are not too long, but I can't read books at all, not even middle grade children's books. At the beginning, I tried to read a guide book by ME/CFS specialist Dr. Sarah Myhill, but never got past the first two chapters, even in tiny installments. Reading requires immense concentration. When I persisted through one chapter of a novel, I became very ill for days.

Even holding a conversation is difficult. My husband only speaks to me on a need-to-know basis. He cannot tell me the myriad tales involving his friends, his house renovation fantasies, or the olfactory delight of discovering and dealing with the blocked drain behind our house. The effort required to follow such idle chit chat drains precious energy. He also cannot start a conversation if I am on my feet, for I can neither wait on my feet to finish the conversation, nor return to finish it, and undertake the task of travelling to another room all over again!

~~~~~~~

I react unpredictably to ordinary stresses. Emotional or psychological strain of any sort literally turns me into jelly. Shouting at the children, a phone call to the insurance company, having to rush for something, and even recounting my awful struggles here makes my whole body feel weak and wobbly, making bed rest a necessary recourse.

This reaction is bewildering. For "activity" relates only to the physical, in most people's minds. However, in ME/CFS, all activity must be taken into account – physical, mental, social, emotional and psychological. Energy usage must be allowed for accordingly, or it runs out.

The clinic gave one explanation which did make some sense. All the stress hormones, such as cortisol and adrenaline, and the resulting increase in metabolic rate, consume a lot of energy. This isn't noticeable when a person is healthy and wakes up with 100 energy chips every day, but has a profound effect when one wakes up with only two!

A fellow patient provided an alternative explanation: "Strong emotions are a form of sensory overload," she said. Just as sound wears me out and a brightly lit room isn't restful, strong emotions simply consume too much brainpower to process.

~~~~~~~

Energy chips – that's how I think of the problem. A normal person wakes up with 100 chips in the morning if they have had a very good night. Most days they will wake up with about 95 chips, or 90 if they've had a very busy week. Even if they were ill or were out drinking until 3 o'clock in the morning, they will not dip below 70 chips.

I wake up with just two to five chips. With this, I have to get through my day. If I have a shower, I use up one chip. Washing my hair doubles that. If

I experience any emotional or psychological stress, another chip or two is spent. Filling in a 50-page social benefit form consumes four chips!

I never know for sure how I am going to be from one day to the next. Making plans is impossible. If I have been doing too much, I wake up with fewer chips. Then I have to spend many hours in bed. When I have a crash, I have to get by on just ONE miserable chip!

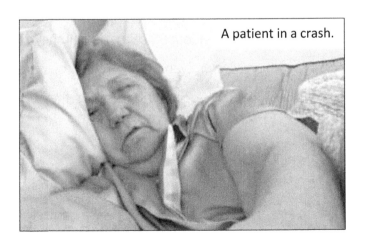
A patient in a crash.

When Mummy is Sick

My little girl has been stuck in the house all day with me. She has already had to watch a DVD while I had a nap. She thinks that is a treat, but now she's dying to go out and play on her balance bicycle.

I am in a Slow Start. I just want to lie on the sofa. Everything is so heavy, such an effort to move. The thought of balancing on a stool, which my husband has bought for this purpose, makes me want to lie down even more!

But I love my child. So I grab some pillows and cushions, and sit down on the curb, leaning against a neighbour's garden wall.

I look odd. Eyebrows rise. When neighbours come out of their homes, I do not go over to chat. I do not have the strength, so I stay firmly on my bottom.

But my daughter is happy. She zooms up and down the street, her little legs going like the clappers. She runs up a neighbour's steep drive, and flies back down on her bicycle, right across the road and into the opposite pavement. She is delighted to show me how fast she can go, and I am thrilled to get to see it.

~~~~~~~

Another day and I don't even have the strength to sit leaning against the wall. So I lay a mat down on my drive, settle with my cushions, and lie down with a cloth over my face. I try to look up every so often to check that my little girl is ok. Fortunately she spends a lot of time cycling in little circles around me. The slope on our drive is fun for her too. I pretend the neighbours think I'm sunbathing, even though no-body does it on their driveway.

Sometimes when I am on my own with her, my little girl says to me, "Mummy, you go and rest now. I want a video."

When I offered to give her her bath one very rare occasion, she asked, "Are you well enough, Mummy?"

~ ~ ~ ~ ~ ~ ~

Today I feel exceptionally good. I take the children to the park. It's only the second time this year, and it's September. The last time, months ago, my husband took us.

The children have been given VERY STRICT instructions not to make it hard for Mummy, when it's time to come home. They understand that if Mummy has to wrestle them into the car, we will not be going again, and if Mummy has to telephone Daddy for help, there will be no chicken for dinner. They agree to anything, for the chance to be out.

~ ~ ~ ~ ~ ~ ~

We go in the car even though the park is just behind our house. I spend the whole time sitting on the bench, flopped over onto the wooden picnic table.

My little girl tries to get into the swing but it's above her head. Her brother, seven years of age, tries to lift her in and fails. I watch and will a nearby parent to lift her in. She doesn't.

They run off and play on the spinning roundabout, then they try again at the swing. This time they succeed. My son gets kicked in the face every time the swing comes back, but he does his best to push his sister. Because I'm not there to supervise, my little girl gets smacked in the face on the rebound when coming off the swing. I watch as she wails in pain.

She pulls herself together and runs off to play again.

She climbs into a tree. She walks on a log and speaks to a group of strangers. After a while, I send her brother to check that she is ok. By this time she is shouting for him. The strangers have left and perhaps she realises she's alone.

I watch as they run together to the zip wire in the distance, her little head temporarily disappearing behind a man-made hill. Later they come back and tell me my son has been pushing my daughter on the zip wire. I don't know how she got onto it. Perhaps that is just as well.

My little girl takes food from strangers. From where I sit, I can see it's another parent. My son sports an alarming bruise on his left cheek, which over the course of the evening, will grow to one and a half inches in size. I tell him he's been very brave, and how proud I am of him for looking after his sister. When it's time to go home, their behaviour is exemplary.

~ ~ ~ ~ ~ ~ ~ ~

Several things happen too close together, and now I am suffering a downturn. I am really not supposed to leave the house at all, and if I do for very rare, special occasions, I must be prepared to pay the price.

I do not make it to the park again this year. The next time I go, nearly six months later, I suffer payback so severe it inspires an essay. After that, I *never* get to the park again.

http://bit.ly/one-at-a-time

Post Exertional Malaise (PEM)

The prolonged worsening of all symptoms, sometimes with emergence of new symptoms or symptoms not normally present, when any activity over a patient's safe limit is attempted.

How Bad Can it Get?

After going off sick, I needed to have a battery of blood tests done. So ignoring the desire for sleep, I drove to the phlebotomist, and sat with my eyes shut in the waiting room. I did not know then what I know now. I felt abnormally tired, but accepted it as part of my likely diagnosis – ME/CFS, not knowing how damaging it was to push through when I needed rest. I thought nothing of driving exhausted, as I had been driving to and from work until just two days before.

That day, I became so ill I couldn't get out of bed. To get to the toilet, I had to lean against the walls, doors and chair, and my knees wobbled from being so weak. Standing up made my head woozy.

It was frightening. I worried it might be Guillain Barre Syndrome (recent multiple severe and systemically debilitating sore throats), or Myasthenia Gravis (fatiguability).

The doctor examined me, testing my muscle power. The effort of flexing my muscles for him left me shaking, even lying in bed, I was so weak. I was left bedridden for two days.

~~~~~~~

There has been multiple crashes. Life seemed to be a cycle of becoming severely debilitated, and then taking six weeks to get just a little strength back. I would then attempt to build myself back up by going for walks round my little cul de sac, only to quickly crash again. Each crash was a crushing disappointment, made harder by the fact that I could not know what to expect. I would think I'd be better after two or three days, but find that I was still just as ill after two weeks.

Over time, I learnt how drastically I must restrict my activities in order to maintain a stable baseline. I also learnt how much energy non-physical things consume. Cold weather, having visitors, and the children being off school all take their toll. Emotional and psychological stresses had to be brought under control.

I learnt to better understand and interpret how I feel. Where early on I would have thought, "I'm feeling lazy today", and proceeded to spend the day doing something sedentary, I now know it means I have done too much, and need complete rest until I feel better, or I will suffer a full crash. That means avoiding even mental exertion, and it does not guarantee I will not crash.

This is a very different mindset for someone who has never before been allowed to "feel lazy"!

~~~~~~~

Once when I crashed, I went five days without a shower. I got out of bed only to eat and to use the bathroom. Getting to the kitchen was a mammoth task. Every step and stumble was a fight, everything hurt, and I felt a hundred years old. Day and night I was in bed, alone. It so happened that everyone had gone to my in-laws' for the week. For that I was grateful, as I did not want my children to see me in such a frightening state.

After so many cycles of crashing and recovering painfully slowly, it was soul-destroying for it to happen yet again, when I had been so careful with my activity levels. I felt I had no control. I was terrified that I would never get better, that I would wither away and die. I was afraid that I would never again be the clever doctor who helps people. I was heartbroken about all the things I couldn't do with my children, and I mourned all the losses if I should die.

After five days, I finally managed to have a shower and wash my hair. I had to do it sitting on the floor, and shampoo my hair twice because it was in such a state. Afterwards, I was so exhausted I had to lie in bed for two hours, desperately trying not to fall asleep, before I gained the strength to brush my hair. Then I couldn't fight it any longer. Sleep took me – I could not brush my teeth.

Thankfully by the end of the week, I had improved a little. I could move like an eighty-year-old instead of a hundred – very slowly, but manageable if I held on to the banister, walls and furniture. Hallelujah! I was relieved that my children didn't have to be frightened to see me when they got home.

~~~~~~~

Four years have passed. Now because I try to be careful how much I do, my crashes are no longer so spectacular. Instead, every time I overdo it or have a stressful experience, I get a little worse and never recover. Over time, I have gradually deteriorated. Going eight or nine days between showers now seems normal, and I have gone as long as sixteen days. Once upon a time not having a shower for five days seemed dreadful.

Over the autumn and winter I had deteriorated, and by April I had not regained my previous function. In the last two weeks, I have crashed yet again, and now I reach a new functional low. If the last setback is anything to go by, it may take me the rest of the year to recover, if I ever do. It is my perpetual dream that with enough rest, I will recover from the latest slide to regain the previous level of function, and from there to gradually improve.

Now I have to rest in bed repeatedly through the day, my sleep pattern is severely deranged, and just standing up causes my heart rate to increase by 30 bpm. I no longer fold the laundry. Any trip out of the house is a major ordeal. I am nauseated from motion sickness and severe light sensitivity. I must wear extremely dark sunglasses and a black towel over my face, and be wheeled around very gently in a wheelchair. I cannot see where I'm going and I look completely insane.

Even within the house, I must wear a varying combination of sunglasses, baseball cap and black towel just to be able to leave my bedroom. Now that I have finally worked out what medical help I could ask for, I am too sick to attend the appointments. For me, the possibility of dying before my children are grown is real. Yet I have an even greater fear. That is, that either of my children should ever be stricken by this cruel, yet unrecognised and neglected illness, and have his or her brimming potential stopped dead in its tracks.

"Patients with ME/CFS have been found to be more functionally impaired than... congestive heart failure... multiple sclerosis... end-stage renal disease"

Institute of Medicine, 2015

Farewell – A Last Post from Anne Örtegren:

http://bit.ly/HR-AnneO-Farewell

My photos:

http://bit.ly/DrHngPhotos

My Take on Sleep

A doctor once said to me that "unrefreshing sleep" is the hallmark of ME/CFS. Having lived through this, I believe it's not that sleep is unrefreshing, but rather that sufferers need so much sleep they just don't get enough to feel refreshed.

In the beginning, I suffered what must have sounded like "unrefreshing sleep" to a doctor. I woke up in the morning feeling shattered, muscles screaming and brain protesting, just as I had felt when I went to bed at night. It was as if the night's sleep hadn't happened, even though it had. Doctors dealing with ME/CFS patients must hear repeatedly, "I feel like I haven't slept at all."

After several months, I started to feel as if I had slept. I still became tired again very quickly, but for a short period after sleeping, I did feel better. And my theory on it is this:

ME/CFS sufferers have a very large sleep deficit and need to catch up on it before sleep starts to feel refreshing.

Put it this way: If you need 200 hours of sleep, eight or ten hours isn't going to make you feel any better. The only answer is to sleep, and sleep some more, until you have caught up.

After a night's sleep, you will have only just clocked up your normal daily requirement under ordinary circumstances, which may be six or seven hours, or as many as nine. That means you may have banked one hour towards your enormous deficit of 200 hours. That is why you need naps in the day and very long nights.

I present this as an alternative perspective on the "unrefreshing sleep". I think it is important because thinking of it this way encourages the right management – sleep your way towards recovery, not just accept it as an inevitable feature of the illness. Perhaps rather than "unrefreshing sleep", it should be called "relatively insufficient sleep"!

I would not be surprised if chronic severe sleep deprivation is eventually found to be a major risk factor for developing ME/CFS, such as that experienced by healthcare workers and shift workers. In my opinion, if you feel like sleeping, you should sleep, whatever the time of day, because you cannot improve until you have rectified your sleep deficit.

As for the much touted advice on "sleep hygiene", I say forget it! Sleep hygiene (a dreadful term, as if sleep is somehow bad or dirty) may be useful for healthy individuals suffering from insomnia, but in ME/CFS, represents no more than guesswork. If arrogance and stubbornness gets in the way of good clinical observation and humility, guesswork can turn into authoritative advice, sometimes with disastrous consequences.

ME/CFS sufferers may need specific help with insomnia, but if the problem is merely a perceived wrong of sleeping or being awake at unconventional times, remember the late Dr. Elizabeth Dowsett, one of the most knowledgeable authorities of her time on ME, always spoke of "living within the rhythm of the brain" while it tries to heal itself.[S]

_____

[S] The Young ME Sufferers Trust "Banned from sleeping"
http://bit.ly/TTBannedFromSleeping

Ripples in a Pond

Such a devastating illness affects EVERYONE around you. From anxiety to grief, anger to understanding, attitudes and priorities to psychological and financial issues, the adjustments are massive. Friends are lost, new friends are made. The world shrinks. Families fall apart.

Your extended family have to pull together. Your colleagues have to fill the gap you leave, and your friends have to accommodate your new "normal". Some people have to be removed from your life altogether!

With ME, there is no choice in the matter. When a person is so draining of energy that just having them as an active contact on your phone, never knowing when a message might come in, turns your body into jelly and your knees into mush, and keeps you bedridden all day, there is no option but to remove that person from your life.

Your home environment and that of all who live with you, or who visit, must be strictly controlled. Noise, light, fragrances, the interior decoration, the bedding, everybody's wardrobes, the entertainment, and even conversation must be adjusted to accommodate. The more severe the illness, the more restrictive life becomes for everyone. Some afflicted parents, tragically, cannot tolerate the presence of their children. ME truly requires saintly levels of awareness and understanding.

If you are lucky, people act with love for your children. But disbelief and dismissal is common. Our illness does not show outwardly, and our disability is invisible. One mother shares her heartbreaking experience with us. The photos that follow show the people most affected by my illness.

Julia's story

"I had three kids and I had no family or friends around. During my bedbound years I would hear the kids whispering outside my bedroom about who was staying off school because I was so ill that day. I was too out of it to speak. We never told anyone, all terrified we would be split up by social services. My kids asking who would look after them if I died. Sometimes I wouldn't see them for weeks at a time, as I would be asleep when they were awake and vice versa. We communicated with written notes.

I had managed the first twelve years of my eldest's life on and off, but the other two were nine and seven when I started going downhill. My eldest left for New Zealand at 18 and the other two were 14 and 12, left to cope with my illness and raise themselves and deal with all things in life on their own including bullying. I feel tremendous guilt that this was their life, no holidays or days at the beach. When I nearly died from organ failure and I could hear my kids crying I was devastated.

I have never met my twin granddaughters who are three, and haven't seen my grandson who is eight, since he was three. Everyone thinks I'm just lazy so attitudes toward me are awful.

My other daughter lives at home and has a two-year-old with autism. She does some cleaning and all the cooking and shopping and the dog walks when I can't manage, but also pays £200 a week in nursery fees as she knows I can't cope. Even just to run to the shop she has to get him dressed because he's an active toddler and I can't look after him. Lots of guilt.

My children have been my carers. This was not why I had kids and not the life I wanted them to have. I haven't parented them, they've parented me. It's like I gave birth to carers."

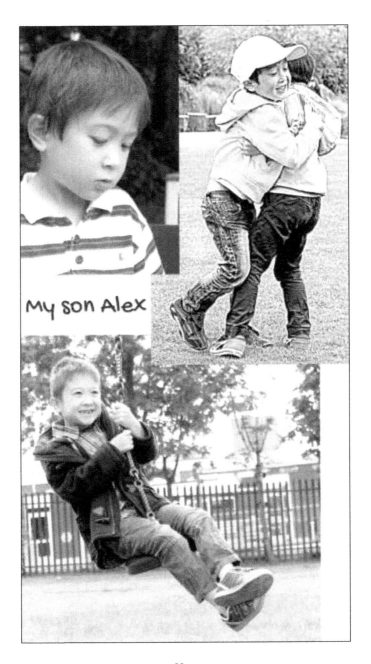

My son Alex

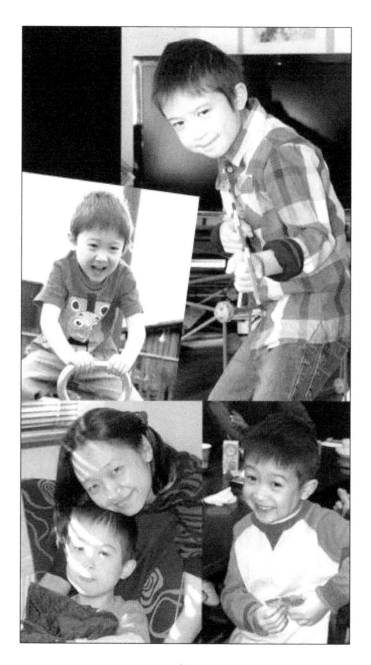

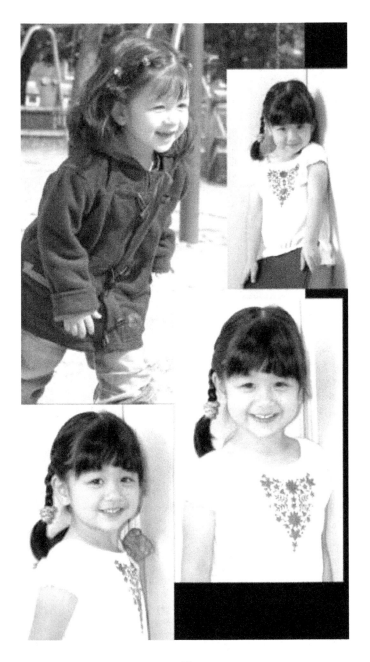

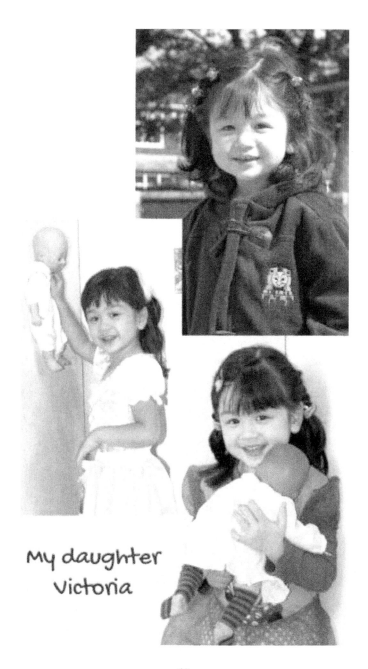

My daughter
Victoria

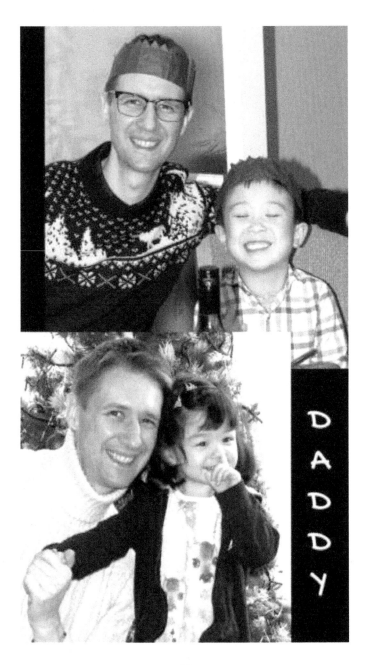

DADDY

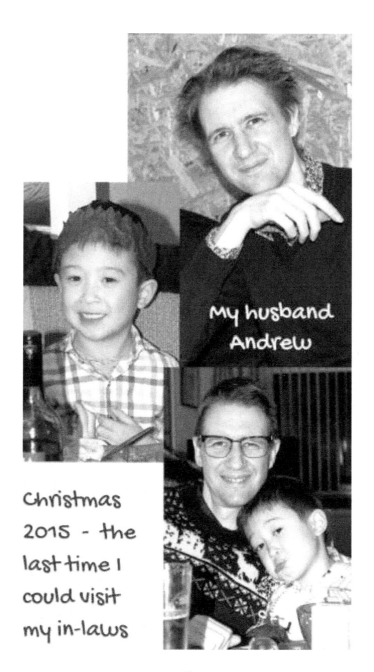

My husband
Andrew

Christmas
2015 - the
last time I
could visit
my in-laws

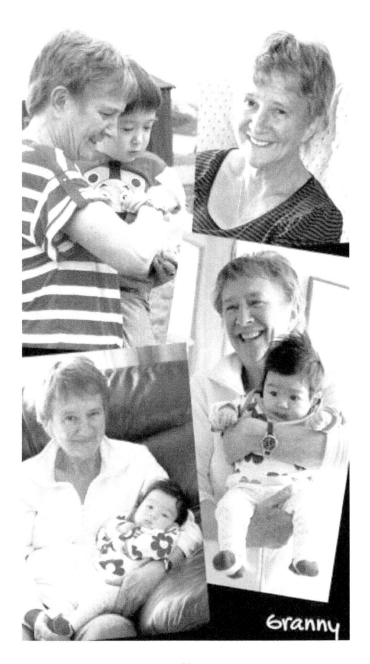

Granny

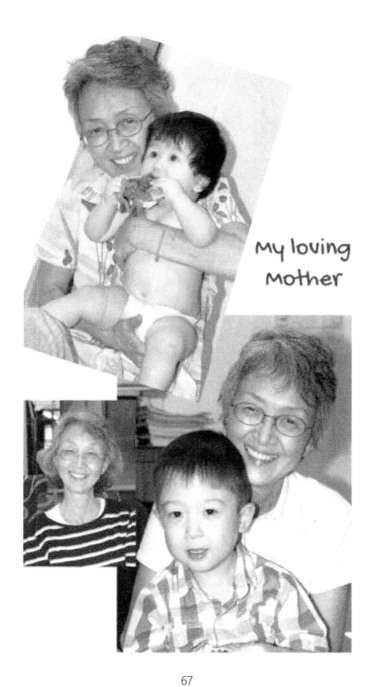

My loving
Mother

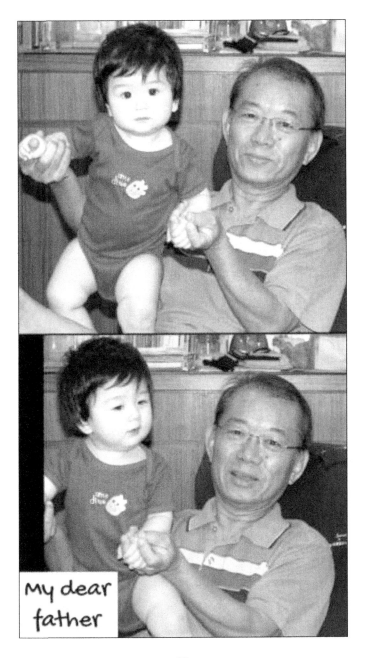

My dear father

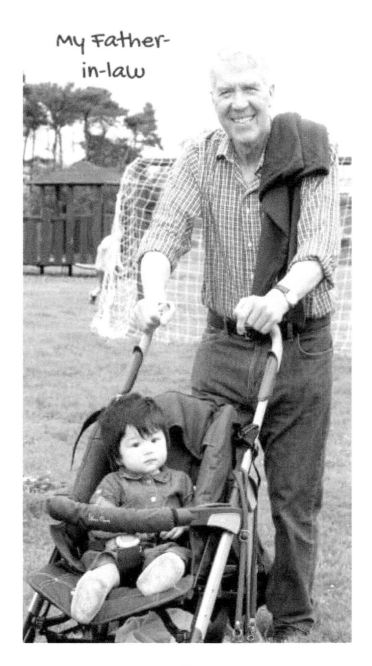

My Father-
in-law

Invisible

When neighbours no longer saw me do my walks around our street, they assumed I had gone back to work. In actual fact I had crashed and was stuck in my bed. At work, despite feeling dreadful, I looked so normal that none of the dozens of doctors I worked with even considered that I might be ill.

Nobody sees us when we are down. When we are better and we do the few things that we can do, be it a little housework or some grocery shopping, we look well, and no one has any idea of the exhaustion that follows, or the hours spent in bed in between.

Many, many moons ago I accompanied my son to the Young Harps workshop at the Royal Northern College of Music. My husband drove, and apart from the last twenty minutes when I watched my son perform with the other children, I spent the morning sleeping on a bench. Even so, upon returning home I had to spend all afternoon in bed, and I didn't brush my teeth at all that day. I also skipped my shower for the third day in a row.

If we have visitors, we rest for days beforehand in preparation, and our visitors see us interacting with them. But once they are gone, we pay the price, taking days or weeks to recover. Again, nobody knows the sacrifice it takes to be able to see our friends once in a blue moon, the debilitation we live with, the choices we make. The world only sees us when we are functional.

I can't remember when I last went to the dentist or the hairdresser. In the end my husband cut my hair at home, for it had grown unmanageable.

Across the globe, thousands of young people spend all their days in quiet, darkened rooms, unable to tolerate any sensory stimulation. Some are unable to even feed themselves, while others move only by dragging their rag doll bodies across the floor in their homes. With decades of unbearable suffering, in severe pain and with no end in sight, many have taken their own lives, and experts report an excess of deaths from cancer and heart failure.[A,B,C]

Yet the medical community is largely ignorant of the magnitude of our suffering, the extent of our disability, the serious and multi-system nature of our illness, the multiplicity of our symptoms, and our physical pain. When we are too unwell we can't get to the doctor, and when we do go to them we look completely normal and all standard tests are negative.

The doctor doesn't see me crawl on the floor. The doctor doesn't know I don't shower every day or brush my teeth twice a day like everyone else. He isn't aware of my frequent sore throats, my poor balance, my difficulties with reading, my muscle twitches, my sound and light intolerance, or the fact that I cannot stand up long enough to have a shower so must do it sitting on the floor. He certainly wasn't here to nurse me when I have been too weak to eat.

The confusing, trivialising and inappropriate name for the condition "Chronic Fatigue Syndrome" further serves to reinforce the impression that there is nothing really wrong. Effectively, we are invisible.

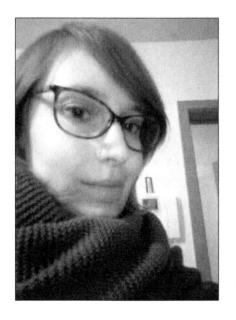

What
people see

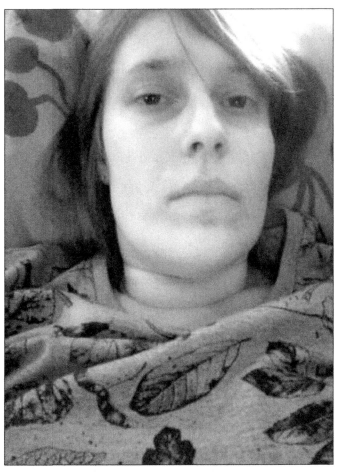

Note the myopathic facies. ME patients are truly sick; such is the extent of our muscle weakness.

What people don't see. This young lady has been sick since the age of 12.

Many patients are misdiagnosed with a psychological illness such as depression or told that it's all in their heads. This is not only unhelpful but actually harmful. It robs patients of the option of the right management, and a psychological approach of "positive thinking", encouraging patients to ignore their symptoms and carry on with activity, or worse, to exercise, is the most harmful intervention possible. The damage can be great and many patients never recover. In the misguided pursuit of psychological or psychiatric cures, some patients are even incarcerated in mental institutions!

The situation is even more shocking with children.[D] Across the country, child protection proceedings are instigated against parents trying to protect their sick children from forced harmful treatments. Accusations of Munchausen by Proxy or Factitious and Induced Illness abound. Some children have been removed from their caring homes and placed into hospitals and institutions where they have been systematically abused by well-meaning professionals intent on forcing them to exercise. Needless to say, these children only get sicker, and are severely traumatised.

http://voicesfromthe shadowsfilm.co.uk/

http://bit.ly/ChldnW mecfsVidMay2018

Rest and pacing of activities is EXTREMELY important in the management of this illness. It is the mainstay of treatment for sadly, even when a patient is taken seriously and given the right diagnosis, there is no effective cure the doctors can offer. For decades this invisible illness has had little attention from the scientific and research community, and our understanding of its causation, let alone potential treatments, is glaringly scant.

Exercise in ME – the science:
http://bit.ly/VoicesGET

A. "Mortality in Patients with Myalgic Encephalomyelitis and Chronic Fatigue Syndrome", by Jason et al.
Fatigue. 2016;4(4):195-207.
https://www.ncbi.nlm.nih.gov/pubmed/28070451

B. "Causes of death among patients with chronic fatigue syndrome", by Jason et al.
Health Care Women Int. 2006 Aug;27(7):615-26.
https://www.ncbi.nlm.nih.gov/pubmed/16844674

C. "Farewell – A Last Post from Anne Örtegren"
http://bit.ly/HR-AnneO-Farewell

D. "False Allegations of Child Abuse in Cases of Childhood Myalgic Encephalomyelitis (ME)"
by Jane Colby, Executive Director of Tymes Trust.
Argument and Critique. July 2014.
http://bit.ly/TTChildAbuse

Solace in Creativity

In my exile, I began to explore my creativity. The children and I played with loom bands and Hama beads. I took photos and videos of them. Before I was properly diagnosed, the Occupational Health doctor had said I had "work related stress", and recommended a healthy dose of child's play! And it really did feel good "wasting time" doing things just because they were fun, like making a whole fleet of multi-coloured seahorses.

At one point, I started playing the piano. It took many, many months of repeated crashes and even-tually learning to remain housebound in order to keep things more stable, before I could do that. I could only play for very short periods. Half an hour would be too long. All my energy would be spent, I would become very weak, start shaking, and have to rest in bed.

I shake because my muscles are unable to maintain a steady posture. My knees wobble and I can't hold myself up. When I lift a hand, it manifests as a tremor. The same thing happens after a game of chess. The mental exertion consumes more energy than can be supplied by my sick mitochondria, so draining the available stores. In other words, I mustn't even *think* too much!

> Mitochondria are the powerhouses within each cell in the body. They burn fuel (sugars, fats) to make energy (ATP molecules).

I am no longer able to play the piano. I dream of the day that I can enjoy it once more, but for now, I must be content with just watching my children's successes, captured on video, especially during the dark hours in bed when I am too weak to move anything but my arms.

After the creative craft toys, my attention turned to the coloured music sheets that I had made for my son over the years. I decided to do them properly on the computer, as I needed more music for the children. Soon I found myself writing some very easy lessons to go with the music, with other parents in mind.

Publication was a pie in the sky, but I carried on, putting my ideas onto paper. I couldn't help myself, for I am a teacher at heart. Teaching was the one area at work in which I still excelled, even as I lived through hell not knowing I was ill.

Now the ideas kept coming. I wrote progressive lessons and arranged the music around them, filling eight books. The teacher in me was calling out. This was such a fun and easy way for beginners to play music, I wanted all children, and any adults who wished they could play, to try it!

There is no need to worry about music lessons. Unlike other music books, my books are meant to be used at home by parents rather than by music teachers. They are a great way to start for anyone uncertain about the commitment to formal lessons. Even for those who never intend to take lessons, they form a large bank of easy fun.

Over time, I managed to get the first three books in the series published. They can be found on Amazon, with the title "Fun Piano for Children", and numbered Book 1, Book 2 and Book 3.

~~ The End ~~

"I split my clinical time between [ME/CFS and HIV], and I can tell you if I had to choose between the two illnesses I would rather have HIV."

Dr. Nancy Klimas

Director, Institute for Neuro Immune Medicine, Nova Southeastern University.

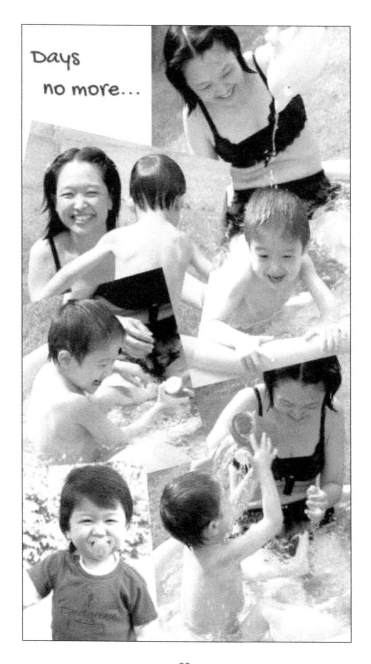

Days
no more…

Medics Corner: Resources

How to diagnose ME:

http://bit.ly/IntConsPrimerME2012

How to rule out other conditions:

http://bit.ly/IACFS-ME-primer-2014

Danger of exercise:

http://bit.ly/EmAus-PEM-GET-2017

Paediatric ME:

https://doi.org/10.3389/fped.2017.00121

CDC website on ME/CFS:

http://bit.ly/CDCme-cfsHP

Medics Corner:
4 videos and a story

Dr. David Kaufman summary:

http://bit.ly/D-KaufmanMEcfs2018

Bateman Horne Center videos:

http://bit.ly/BHC-mecfs

Mitochondria not Hypochondria cartoon:

http://bit.ly/MitoNotHypo

Paediatric ME:

http://bit.ly/SpeightRoweVids2018

A story: **http://bit.ly/TheTerribleTale**
OfAmyBrown

Critical Review:
Graded Exercise Therapy for ME/CFS

- Studies were done in high functioning patients who may not have had ME/CFS. Therefore not applicable to patients who are house or bed bound.

- Broad entry criteria not requiring Post Exertional Malaise, an essential diagnostic criteria for ME.

- Inadequate reporting of harms and high dropout rate means GET cannot be assumed to be safe. Patient surveys report very high rates of harm (60-82%).

- Subjective outcomes highly prone to bias.

- Objective outcomes show GET is ineffective in the treatment of ME/CFS.

http://bit.ly/GET-crit-rv-MarkVink

Critical Review:

Cognitive Behavioural Therapy for CFS/ME

- Most studies were on patients well enough to attend clinic, including some with near normal function. Not applicable to patients who are housebound.

- Broad entry criteria include a large proportion of patients with psychiatric morbidity and patients who may not have ME.

- Subjective outcomes highly prone to bias.

- Only one in seven patients report a small, short-lived, subjective reduction in fatigue.

- No improvement in objective measures such as physical fitness, benefits status or hours worked.

- One in five patients come to harm.

http://bit.ly/CBT-crit-rv-MarkVink

Medics Corner: A crystal ball

Will my patient be fit for work again?

Literature review:
Work Rehabilitation and Medical Retirement for ME/CFS Patients

http://bit.ly/Vink-WorkRehab-MedRetirement

Summary:

http://bit.ly/WorkRehab2019

"The fact that Dr. Hng had to suffer for so long before being diagnosed is a serious reflection on current medical education in the UK.

Despite being a doctor herself, and quite far on in her medical career, and having the MRCP and being a medical teacher, she had clearly been deprived of sufficient knowledge of ME to be able to diagnose herself. This reflects the virtual denial of the reality of ME with which much of the UK medical profession currently treats the condition."

Dr. Nigel Speight

Consultant Paediatrician and ME specialist

Epilogue

A NEW PURPOSE

When I first put pen to paper, my vision was to make available a book which will show doctors what it really is to be ill with Myalgic Encephalomyelitis. I wanted doctors to realise that this is a real illness, it is not at all trivial, and it is not of psychological origin. I wanted patients to know that their suffering is real, and that they are not imagining it. And I wanted to give sufferers a way of explaining to others what it is that is wrong with them, and for them to be believed by their family and friends, to be understood.

To this end I strove simply to make the book available on Amazon. As a complete novice to the world of writing and publishing, and with limited energy, this seemed a satisfactory goal to me. How wrong I was!

In the process of writing this book, communicating with other sufferers, reading around the subject, and connecting with advocates and experts, I have learnt so much. As soon as the book was released, I realised this was not the end, but just the beginning. It was the beginning of a lifelong mission of education and advocacy. Like thousands of other patients before me, many much sicker than I am, it is my fate to join the fight for proper recognition and treatment, on behalf of those who cannot fight for themselves.

I now run a large international Facebook group where I educate, advocate and support. Readers are invited to join me. The group is called **Dr Hng's ME/CFS Friends.**

Much goes on in the online world. There is a role to suit every individual, however much or little energy one can spare. Group members have produced an amazing album of original music and poetry, written and performed by ME patients and their families from all over the world. A sample of our offerings can be seen here: **http://bit.ly/Music4MEpageFB** To purchase the album or donate towards medical education on ME, see details on pages 4 and 5.

To reach as many people as possible, this book has been translated into Czech, French and Polish, and other translations are underway. We are also working on audio and electronic versions. I hope that over time, many other languages will be added.

Behind the scenes, I work with others to explore options in medical education. If you think you can help, please get in touch.

We are sick, but we are many. Together, we will bring change and improve the situation. Join us!

Motion passed in UK Parliament 24/1/2019

This house:

- Calls on the Government to provide increased funding for biomedical research for the diagnosis and treatment of ME.

- Supports the suspension of Graded Exercise Therapy and Cognitive Behaviour Therapy as means of treatment.

- Supports updated training of GPs and medical professionals to ensure that they are equipped with clear guidance on the diagnosis of ME and appropriate management advice to reflect international consensus on best practice.

- Is concerned about the current trends of subjecting ME families to unjustified child protection procedures.

http://bit.ly/MEdebateJan2019H

Afterword

IT'S ALL IN YOUR HEAD

ME or CFS?

The correct name for my illness is Myalgic Encephalomyelitis (ME). Chronic Fatigue Syndrome (CFS) is not a diagnosis, but a collection of symptoms. It does not represent one specific disease entity. Some CFS diagnostic criteria specifically exclude the more severe of ME symptoms, or do not require the cardinal ME symptom of Post-Exertional Neuroimmune Exhaustion (PENE, also known as Post Exertional Malaise, PEM) – that is, the worsening of all symptoms after any over-activity. In effect, cases of ME can be excluded in a CFS diagnosis, and the lack of specificity means patients with fatigue from a multitude of other causes can be diagnosed with CFS.

Therefore, while many CFS patients actually have ME, being handed a diagnosis of CFS is in truth to be told, "You meet these criteria so we will say you have CFS but we haven't really diagnosed what's actually wrong with you." Chronic Fatigue Syndrome is thus a non-diagnosis.

In many parts of the world, ME is not recognised and only the term CFS is used. The two names are also frequently stuck together in various permutations. There is a sense that after the non-diagnosis Chronic Fatigue Syndrome was invented, ME was pulled into the mix as a fatiguing illness, so that it no longer needed to be treated as a serious physical illness, but merely a psychological or psychosomatic one.[1] Many believe this was intentional – it has had significant impact on social benefit bills and insurance payouts. This conflation of names has become so widespread, that in practice it is often difficult to drop the term CFS without excluding patients from receiving proper care.

The incorrect use of the term CFS as a synonym for ME, and the irresponsible promotion of psychological treatments for "CFS/ME" in official guidelines, has caused a lack of understanding among clinicians, and persuaded people that ME is a psychological condition. Research using CFS diagnostic criteria has produced meaningless results which have unfortunately still become the basis for forcing psychological treatments onto ME patients.   However Cognitive Behavioural Therapy (CBT), aimed at "challenging unhelpful beliefs",[2] and Graded Exercise Therapy (GET)[3] are ineffective in ME.[4-7]   Indeed they are dangerous.[6-11]   [Ref 1 pg. 88-97]

Myalgic Encephalomyelitis is not a psychological or mental illness, a neurosis, or behavioural problem. It is an organic disease, with identifiable and measurable pathology. It is in fact a serious multi-system neuro-immune condition.[12-19]   [Ref 1 pg. 5, 98-221]

The gold standard diagnostic criteria for ME is the

2011 International Consensus Criteria (ICC), subse-
quently developed into a Primer.[13] The 2015 Institute
of Medicine (IOM) diagnostic criteria is also gaining
in popularity due to its simplicity.[14] In making a
diagnosis of ME, it is important to rule out other
possible causes of symptoms, as there is currently no
easy diagnostic test for it.[15] The two day Cadiopul-
monary Exercise Test identifies the characteristic Post
Exertional Malaise of ME, but its use is not without its
problems.

One of the most influential, yet most non-specific
and meaningless, diagnostic criteria for Chronic
Fatigue Syndrome is the 1991 Oxford criteria,[20] which
expressly excludes organic brain disease (thus excluding ME) and includes some psychiatric disorders.
Clearly, results of any research based on this loose
definition cannot be applied to ME patients, and
indeed The Agency for Healthcare Research and
Quality (AHRQ) and the National Institutes of Health
(NIH) recommended in 2014 that the Oxford defini-

tion be retired from use in future research.[21,22]

For a better understanding of this complex issue, here is an eye-opening piece of investigative journalism:

http://bit.ly/TullerWorsThanTheDis [23]

Also available is an in-depth analysis into the politics of distorted research, published by the Centre for Welfare Reform in 2016.[24] In addition, Emeritus Professor of Medicinal Chemistry Malcolm Hooper's "MAGICAL MEDICINE: HOW TO MAKE A DISEASE DISAPPEAR" from 2010 is a detailed and thoroughly shocking report.[1]

http://bit.ly/InTheExpOfRecovery [24]

http://bit.ly/MagicalMedicine2010 [1]

Just think positive!

Even in the present day, psychological "treatments" are being actively developed and promoted for CFS/ME, which tell patients to think their symptoms away, alarmingly encouraging them to push beyond their limits, and blaming the patients themselves for not trying hard enough, when they worsen or do not improve!

In Britain and Europe, the psychological narrative sticks tenaciously in official guidelines, clinical research, and many specialist services. Medical education largely ignores the existence of ME altogether! Meanwhile, in the face of medical impotence, expensive commercial "treatments" prey on the desperate and vulnerable. This ranges from miracle supplements to pseudo-scientific psychobabble.

I urge all my readers to be extremely wary of any

treatment which uses a mind over matter approach and tells you not to listen to your body. Even where clinical trial data is cited, I urge you to examine the evidence for yourself and read widely about a proposed treatment before making your decision. Ask yourself the following questions about any clinical trial:

1. Did they recruit the right patients? Or is their entry criteria so loose that they could have recruited patients who actually have depression or anxiety rather than ME? Remember many conditions can cause the "six months of fatigue" used in weak diagnostic criteria for CFS, and any clinical trials using the meaningless Oxford criteria is not applicable to ME patients.

2. Where did the study patients come from? Were they a captive audience that could have been easily manipulated, for example patients attending the clinic of the chief investigator who

hopes to gain financially from a particular treatment? Is there a selection bias? For example, if
only a minority of the patients approached
agreed to participate in a study, what separates
those who agreed and those who did not? The
difference could be that some are ME patients
(though perhaps labelled as having CFS, CFS/ME,
or some other combined name) who know from
experience that a proposed treatment would be
harmful, while others are actually "fatigue"
patients who may have a large psychological
component or other factors.

3. What is the endpoint being studied? For example, this could mean return to work, improvement in function, or psychological effects. Is it an
   objective, measurable endpoint, or a subjective,
   self-reported one? The latter is completely
   meaningless when a psychological approach or
   brainwashing method is being studied (e.g. CBT),
   where participants are programmed to report

positive answers.

4. Did the study measure the originally intended endpoints, or were the goalposts moved before the study was reported?

5. If a trial reports a positive result, is it truly a positive result for ME, or is it inapplicable to ME because of meaningless entry criteria (see point 1) and selection bias (see point 2)? Is the chosen endpoint a meaningful one (see point 3)? And is the result based on the originally chosen end point (see point 4), or merely a modified version that was designed to produce a positive result?

6. And finally, is there any potential conflict of interest, such as a commercial treatment which costs large sums of money, or investigators who also work for insurance companies? Sadly, not all conflicts of interest are properly declared to study participants or in the final publications.

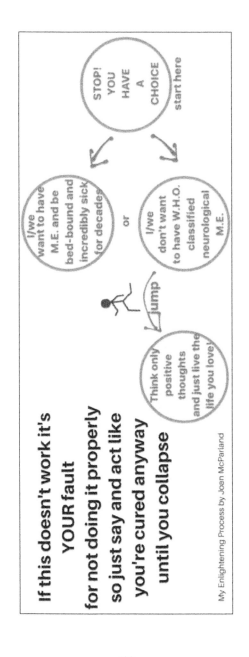

My Enlightening Process by Joan McParland

In your worst interest

At the centre of the great controversy that is ME/CFS is the landmark **PACE** trial,[25,1] published in the Lancet in 2011 and said to be responsible for the recommendation of CBT and GET to ME patients in clinical guidelines all over the world.[26] It is now used as a case study on bad science at the University of California, Berkeley. In February 2018 it was discussed in a UK Parliamentary debate as "one of the biggest medical scandals of the 21st century".[27]

> Watch the PACE debate here:
>
> **http://bit.ly/2oi5b1t**

Rather than showing that CBT and GET are effective treatments for ME, when raw data from the PACE trial, which used the Oxford criteria for CFS, was reanalysed by independent researchers, it was shown that neither are effective treatments, even for Chronic Fatigue Syndrome.[4]   It is noteworthy that said data required a prolonged Freedom of Information legal battle to extract, the attempt to block its release costing the taxpayer a further £245,745 in legal fees,[28] in addition to the £5 million already spent on the trial.[27]   The PACE trial was the only clinical trial to have been part funded by the Department for Work and Pensions.[1 pg.4,19]

Eminent psychologist Prof. Brian Hughes and public health journalist Dr. David Tuller explain the serious problems with the PACE trial here:

What's wrong with the PACE trial?

http://bit.ly/HughesTuller VidOct2018

Numerous other clinical trials attempt to prove and promote the establishment-preferred psychological or exercise treatments. They are fraught with methodological and even ethical flaws. Listed here are some examples, with their disturbing critiques:

The **FINE** trial on "pragmatic rehabilitation":
- http://bit.ly/TullerFINE
- https://phoenixrising.me/archives/11854
- https://bit.ly/2GVKsqE

GETSET on graded exercise:
- https://bit.ly/2KrjUQP
- http://bit.ly/TullerGETSET

The **SMILE** trial on the Lightning Process:
- https://bit.ly/2HGwE4e
- https://bit.ly/2HYTDLz
- https://bit.ly/2IQGjsT

Alleged General Medical Council complaint against

SMILE researcher, source unknown, facts unverified:

- http://bit.ly/SmileRisksPatientEvidence
- http://bit.ly/SmileIllegalTrading
- http://bit.ly/SmileUseChldnNotJstfd

The **University of Bristol** which was involved with the SMILE trial is now running two other studies, on *children* – the **FITNET-NHS** and **MAGENTA** studies. Dr. David Tuller comments:

- http://bit.ly/TullerFITNETnhsNov2016
- http://bit.ly/TullerFollowupFITNETNHS

The situation is similar across Europe, and this manipulation of science has been going on for decades:

- https://bit.ly/2I0Gce7
- http://bit.ly/MagicalMedicine2010
  (pg. 36-43)

While money is endlessly being spent pursuing this nonsense, including this new "shopping bag study" at the **University of Bath**, biomedical research into the causation, disease mechanisms and treatments in ME/CFS struggles for funding.

- https://bit.ly/2rbGvYL
- https://bit.ly/2HGtE8e

Now, as if in desperation from the lack of efficacy thus far, another CBT study recruits *couples* living with CFS:

"...it is believed that involving partners in a constructive manner in a psychological intervention for patients affected by CFS could enhance the effectiveness of the intervention..."

http://bit.ly/2t5tmSL

Are patients' partners and spouses now to be trained to extend the psychological abuse already being levelled at them by their health service, into their homes??

A song by ME/CFS patients from around

the world. Hear our voices:

http://bit.ly/Blowg-in

theWindMEvid

"I have a wish and a dream that medical and scientific societies will apologise to their ME patients."

Dr. Jose Montoya

Professor of Medicine,
Stanford University Medical Centre

Fabricated or Induced Illness /
school phobia / Pervasive Refusal Syndrome?

http://bit.ly/TTChildAbuse

STOP THE HARM

http://bit.ly/ProtectYrself-1

References

1. MAGICAL MEDICINE: HOW TO MAKE A DISEASE DISAPPEAR

   Malcolm Hooper, online booklet, Feb 2010.

   http://bit.ly/MagicalMedicine2010

2. Manual for Therapists COGNITIVE BEHAVIOUR THERAPY for CFS/ME

   Mary Burgess and Trudie Chalder, PACE Trial Management Group.

   http://me-pedia.org/images/b/b4/PACE-cbt-therapist-manual.pdf

3. Manual For Therapists GRADED EXERCISE THERAPY FOR CFS/ME

   Bavinton J, Darbishire L, White PD, PACE Trial Management Group.

   https://me-pedia.org/images/8/89/PACE-get-therapist-manual.pdf

4. Rethinking the treatment of chronic fatigue syndrome – A reanalysis and evaluation of findings from a recent major trial of graded exercise and

CBT

Wilshire et al., *BMC Psychology (2018) 6:6*.
http://bit.ly/PACEre-analysed2018

5. No 'Recovery' in PACE Trial, New Analysis Finds
Vincent Racaniello, *Virology Blog*, 21 Sep 2016.
http://www.virology.ws/2016/09/21/no-recovery-in-pace-trial-new-analysis-finds/

6. Graded exercise therapy for myalgic encephalo-myelitis/chronic fatigue syndrome is not effective and unsafe. Re-analysis of a Cochrane review
Mark Vink and Alexandra Vink-Niese, *Health Psychology Open, July-December 2018: 1–12*.
http://bit.ly/GET-crit-rv-MarkVink

7. Cognitive behavioural therapy for myalgic ence-phalomyelitis/chronic fatigue syndrome is not effective. Re-analysis of a Cochrane review
Mark Vink and Alexandra Vink-Niese, *Health Psychology Open, January-June 2019: 1–23*
http://bit.ly/CBT-crit-rv-MarkVink

8. Opposition to Graded Exercise Therapy (GET) for ME/CFS

VanNess et al., letter to health care providers, 2018.
http://bit.ly/2s7zYms

9. ME/CFS Illness Management Survey Results "No decisions about me without me"
The ME Association, May 2015.
http://bit.ly/MEAssSurvey2015

10. Myalgic encephalomyelitis / chronic fatigue syndrome patients' reports of symptom changes following cognitive behavioural therapy, graded exercise therapy and pacing treatments: Analysis of a primary survey compared with secondary surveys
Geraghty, Hann and Kurtev, *Journal of Health Psychology, 29 Aug 2017.*
http://journals.sagepub.com/eprint/hWSxVIBTz DtqisvafkhE/full

11. Reporting of Harms Associated with Graded Exercise Therapy and Cognitive Behavioural Therapy in Myalgic Encephalomyelitis/Chronic Fatigue Syndrome
Bulletin of the IACFS/ME, 2011;19(2): 59-111.
https://www.iacfsme.org/assets/Reporting-of-Harms-Associated-with-GET-and-CBT-in-ME-

CFS.pdf

12. Centers for Disease Control and Prevention ME/CFS website
http://bit.ly/CDCme-cfsHP

13. MYALGIC ENCEPHALOMYELITIS – Adult & Paediatric: International Consensus Primer for Medical Practitioners
Carruthers et al., online booklet, 2012.
http://bit.ly/IntConsPrimerME2012

14. Beyond Myalgic Encephalomyelitis/Chronic Fatigue Syndrome: Redefining an Illness.
Institute of Medicine, online publication, Feb 2015.
https://www.ncbi.nlm.nih.gov/books/NBK2742 35/

15. Chronic Fatigue Syndrome Myalgic Encephalomyelitis Primer for Clinical Practitioners 2014 Edition
International Association for Chronic Fatigue Syndrome / Myalgic Encephalomyelitis (IACFS/ME), online booklet.
http://bit.ly/IACFS-ME-primer-2014

16. Myalgic Encephalomyelitis / Chronic Fatigue Syndrome Diagnosis and Management in Young People: A Primer
Rowe et al., *Frontiers in Paediatrics, Vol 5, Art 121, June 2017.*
https://doi.org/10.3389/fped.2017.00121

17. Solve ME/CFS Initiative
https://solvecfs.org/

18. Emerge Australia
https://www.emerge.org.au/

19. The National Alliance for Myalgic Encephalomyelitis
https://web.archive.org/web/20180712184807/
http://www.name-us.org/

20. A report – chronic fatigue syndrome: guidelines for research
Sharpe et al., *Journal of the Royal Society of Medicine, Volume 84, pg. 118-121.* February 1991.
https://bit.ly/2I2SORO

21. Diagnosis and Treatment of Myalgic Encephalo-myelitis / Chronic Fatigue Syndrome

    Smith et al., *Evidence Report / Technology Assessment No. 219*. December 2014.
    http://bit.ly/AHRQmecfs2014

22. Pathways to Prevention Workshop: Advancing the Research on Myalgic Encephalomyelitis/ Chronic Fatigue Syndrome, Executive Summary.

    National Institutes of Health, online publication, December 2014.
    http://bit.ly/NIH-mecfs-Research-2014

23. Worse Than the Disease

    David Tuller, *Undark: Truth, Beauty, Science*. 27 Oct 2016.
    http://bit.ly/TullerWorsThanTheDis

24. "In the Expectation of Recovery" MISLEADING MEDICAL RESEARCH AND WELFARE REFORM

    George Faulkner, Centre for Welfare Reform, online booklet, April 2016.
    http://bit.ly/InTheExpOfRecovery

25. Comparison of adaptive pacing therapy, cognitive behaviour therapy, graded exercise therapy, and specialist medical care for chronic fatigue syndrome (PACE): a randomised trial
    White et al., *Lancet; 377: 823–365.* 5 March 2011.
    https://doi.org/10.1016/S0140-6736(11) 60096-2

26. Ethical classification of ME/CFS in the United Kingdom
    Diane O'Leary, *Bioethics;* 2019;00:1–7.
    https://doi.org/10.1111/bioe.12559

27. PACE Trial: People with ME
    House of Commons Hansard, Volume 636. 20 February 2018.
    http://bit.ly/PACEtrial

28. Major breakthrough on PACE trial
    George Faulkner, Centre for Welfare Reform, news article, 19 August 2016.
    http://www.centreforwelfarereform.org/news/ major-breaktn-pace-trial/00296.html

Acknowledgements

I am grateful to my editor Milton Trachtenburg. Thank you also to all the people who have proof-read, commented, provided resources or in some way influenced the book.

Special thanks to Lenka Goldšmídová for translating the book into Czech, Corinne Bourvon for translating it into French, Joanna Osesik for the Polish transla-tion, and the **CFS-ME Organizzazione di Volontariato** for providing the Italian translation. My gratitude to Jacqueline Cox for recording the audio book, to Julia for sharing your experience as a parent with ME, to Joan McParland for your eye-opening depiction of your "Enlightening Process", and to Nathalie Van Eynde and another sick patient, for your photo-graphs.

Thanks as well to many, many other individuals and organisations, including Nigel and Michelle Henshaw, Sharleen Harty, Janice Johnson, my Facebook admin team, contributors to our music fundraiser, and colleagues who collaborate on medical education. You all know how you help the cause.

Finally, my sincere thanks to the **Irish ME/CFS Association** and **Hope 4 M.E. & Fibromyalgia Northern Ireland**, who have purchased books for distribution to members of the medical profession.

Together we are educating people all over the world. Together, we will make a difference!

About the Author

Dr. Hng is a Gastroenterology trainee in the United Kingdom. Her credentials includes her basic medical degree MBChB, 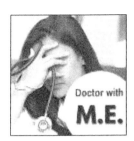 Membership of the Royal College of Physicians (MRCP), Postgraduate Certificate in Work Based Medical Education (PGCert in WBME), and Fellowship of the Higher Education Academy (FHEA).

Dr. Hng excels as a teacher. She was previously a Teaching Fellow, and later an Honorary Lecturer, at the Manchester Medical School, the largest in the country. She is the named author of its Year 3 Liver, Biliary and Pancreatic Diseases online module. Despite her struggle with this debilitating illness, Dr. Hng now attempts the greatest teaching challenge of her life – educating the medical profession on Myalgic Encephalomyelitis!

Made in the USA
Middletown, DE
13 November 2021

52342283R00070